Authentically YOU

A Therapeutic Workbook To Self-Acceptance

Edited by: Keitorria Edmonds – www.TheFinalEdit.CO

Graphics: John Jorif – jjorif@gmail.com

Formatting & Design: Ya Ya Ya Creative – YaYaYaCreative@gmail.com

ISBN: 979-8-9858172-0-1

PRINTED AND BOUND IN THE UNITED STATES OF AMERICA

Table of Contents

This action-oriented, step by step workbook aims to help you achieve self-acceptance and self-love through your self-discovery journey.

What to expect:

- Identify who you are through self-discovery

- Learn all parts of you through self-awareness

- Conquer self-doubt, insecurities, and limitations

- Achieve self-acceptance and self-love

- Live your life being *Authentically You*

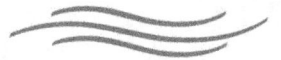

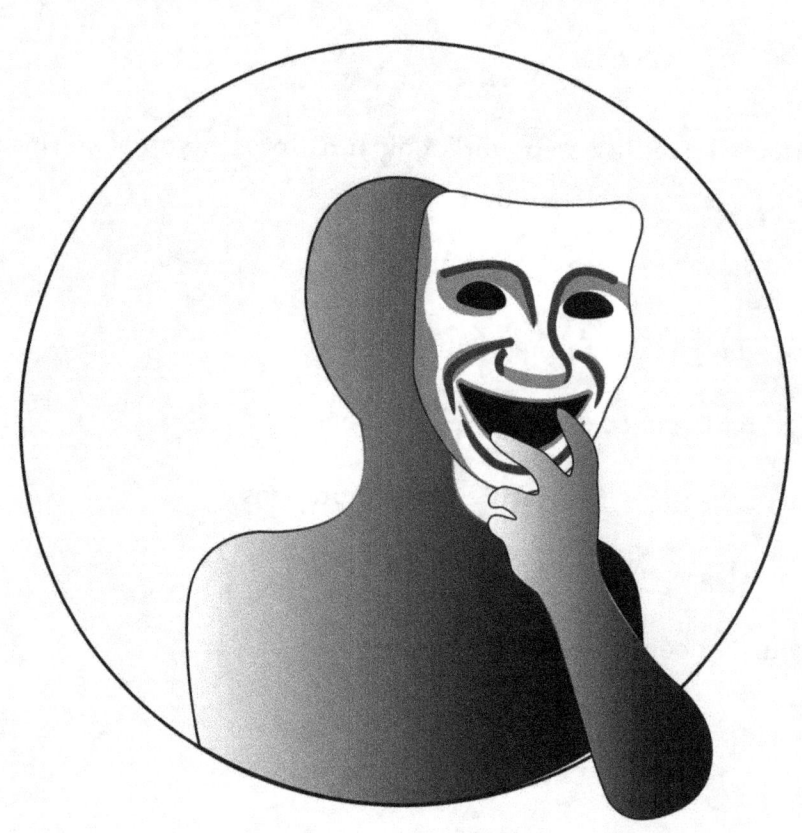

Introduction

The first step to achieving self-acceptance is getting to know who you are. So many times, people put on a mask or façade when interacting with others out of fear of rejection. You feel overwhelmed or uncomfortable about being yourself.

Self-acceptance means showing up without the mask. It means you allow yourself to love everything about you and invite others to know and love you, too. Just imagine living your life with the freedom of not worrying about what others think about you. Imagine no longer making yourself into what you think others will accept.

This does not mean that you do not want to improve areas in your life. Self-acceptance is not an excuse for contentment. There is still work to do. Simply put, it is that you have accepted who you currently are, and you will do the work to reach your goals.

What happens when you achieve self-acceptance?
You accept yourself unconditionally.
Improved self-esteem and confidence.
You will validate yourself.
You liberate yourself from worry.
Your decisions will not be made to please others.
Increased self-awareness.
You will be authentic to yourself and in relationships.

*Before you can truly have
self-acceptance, you must know who you
are. This is learned through self-discovery.
As you utilize this workbook it will take you
on your self-discovery journey. Through your
journey you will become aware of all parts of you.
And therefore, honesty to yourself as you
complete each exercise is imperative to becoming
self-aware, and hopefully, being open to doing any
healing work to accept yourself with unconditional love.*

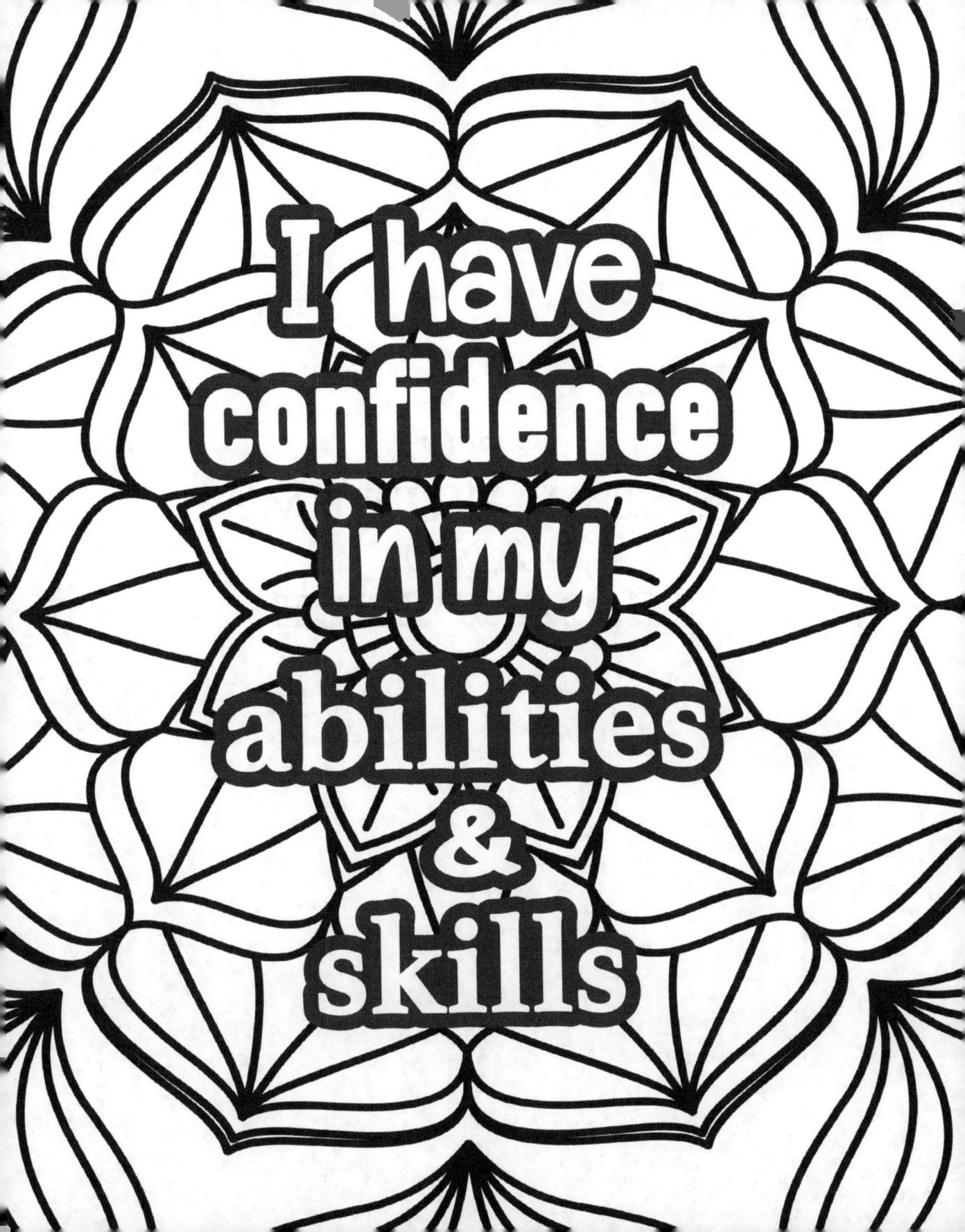

Chapter 1

SELF-ESTEEM AND CONFIDENCE

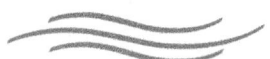

Self-esteem and confidence play a key role on your road to self-acceptance. How you view yourself and your abilities significantly impact being okay with who you are. When you choose self-acceptance, it does not mean you stop caring about the opinions of people that matter to you. In fact, when you accept who you are, you share your own views and opinions more freely. Loving all parts of you, even the ones you want to change, is an important part of this process. Therefore, it is imperative you start off by understanding what self-esteem and confidence are, how these traits develop, and ways to improve your self-esteem and confidence if you struggle in these areas.

What are self-esteem and confidence, and where do they come from?

Self-esteem is confidence in one's own worth, abilities, or morals. Self-esteem encompasses beliefs about oneself (for example, "I am loved", "I am worthy") as well as emotional states, such as triumph, despair, pride, and shame (wikipedia.com)

Self-esteem changes throughout our lives. Our experiences with different people and activities, our childhood, our life's successes and failures, healthy and unhealthy relationships with our family, teachers, authority figures and peers all contribute to the creation of our self-esteem.

Confidence is our self-assurance in trusting our abilities, capacities and judgements; the belief that you can achieve your goals and to be confident in what you have done is okay. (dictionary.com)

Confidence is based on your beliefs about your ability to perform a task successfully. We may be confident in our ability to cook a family meal but have no confidence in our ability to paint a picture. It is based on our experiences.

Healthy Self-Esteem

When you have a healthy self-esteem, you can:

- Acknowledge your strengths and weaknesses and still feel worthy.
- Confidently make decisions.
- Consistently express your needs and opinions.
- Form secure and honest relationships.
- Honestly evaluate yourself and accept the results.

Unhealthy Self-Esteem

When you have an unhealthy self-esteem, often you:

- Feel guilty about your everyday actions.
- Feel undeserving of, or incapable of, having more.
- Have difficulty making your own choices.
- Have difficulty speaking up and prioritizing your own needs, wants, and feelings.
- Lack boundaries in your relationships.

Examples of how healthy self-esteem is formed:

- Being listened to.
- Being spoken to respectfully.
- Being supported and validated.
- Encouragement to pursue goals.

Examples of how unhealthy self-esteem is formed:

- Being harshly criticized.
- Being physically, sexually, or emotionally abused.
- Being ignored, ridiculed or teased.
- Being expected to be perfect all the time.
- Given messages from parents, teachers, authority figures, or peers that failed experiences were failures for the whole self.

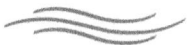

Ways to Build Healthy Self-Esteem and Confidence

Speak positively to yourself

Challenge negative self-talk

Don't compare yourself to others

Acknowledge the positive/ give yourself praise

Write yourself a positive message daily

Practice self-compassion

Take care of your mind, body, and spirit

Be open to try new things

Face your fears

Surround yourself with positive people

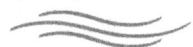

Now that you have an understanding about self-esteem and confidence, rate your self-esteem and confidence on a scale from 1-5. What are some experiences from your life that led to your rating?

| 1 | 2 | 3 | 4 | 5 |

_____

_____

_____

_____

_____

_____

_____

_____

_____

_____

_____

_____

Now that you have learned what has contributed to your level of confidence and self-esteem, what are some things that you plan on doing to build your confidence? Think about what has been discussed in the prior pages.

_____

_____

_____

_____

_____

_____

_____

_____

_____

_____

_____

_____

_____

_____

Twenty-One Days of Building Self-Confidence

Day 1	Day 2	Day 3	Day 4	Day 5	Day 6	Day 7
Do not compare yourself to others	Focus on your strengths	Ditch perfectionism	Challenge your negative thoughts and replace with positive	Smile and make eye contact with others	Set achievable goals for yourself	Prioritize self-discipline and commitment
Day 8	**Day 9**	**Day 10**	**Day 11**	**Day 12**	**Day 13**	**Day 14**
Talk to someone new	Be true to yourself	Sit up and make sure your posture is straight	Speak up and share your opinion	Practice self-care	Write five self-confidence affirmations	Try something new, dive into what you fear
Day 15	**Day 16**	**Day 17**	**Day 18**	**Day 19**	**Day 20**	**Day 21**
Look in the mirror and tell yourself, "I am proud of you and who you are becoming"	Celebrate yourself today	Surround yourself with positive and motivating people and friends	Wear an outfit / attire that makes you feel comfortable and good about yourself	Create a self-esteem collage, include images that represent your positive attributes	Look in the mirror and say, "I love you"	Be kind to yourself and write down three things you are grateful for

_____

_____

_____

_____

_____

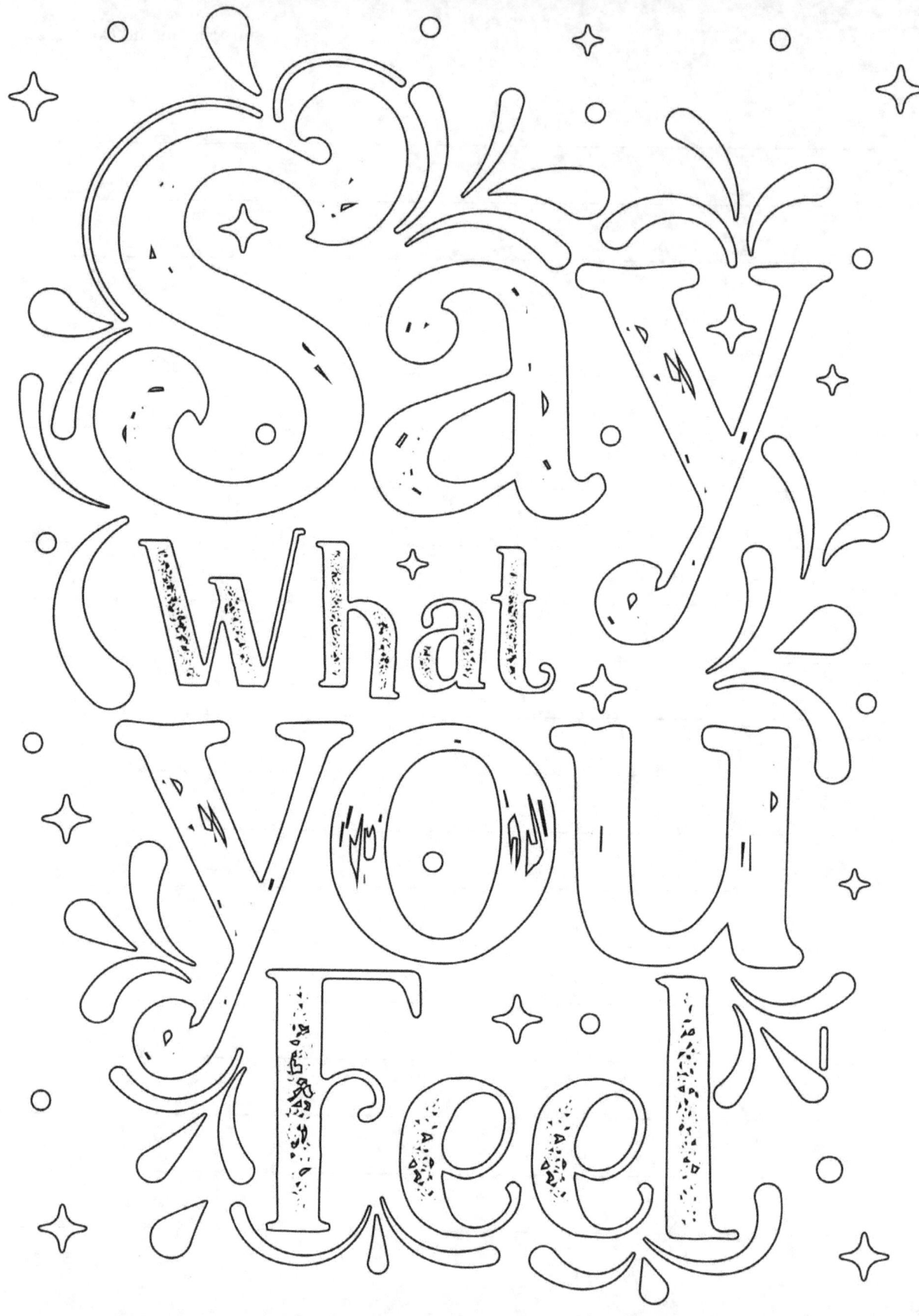

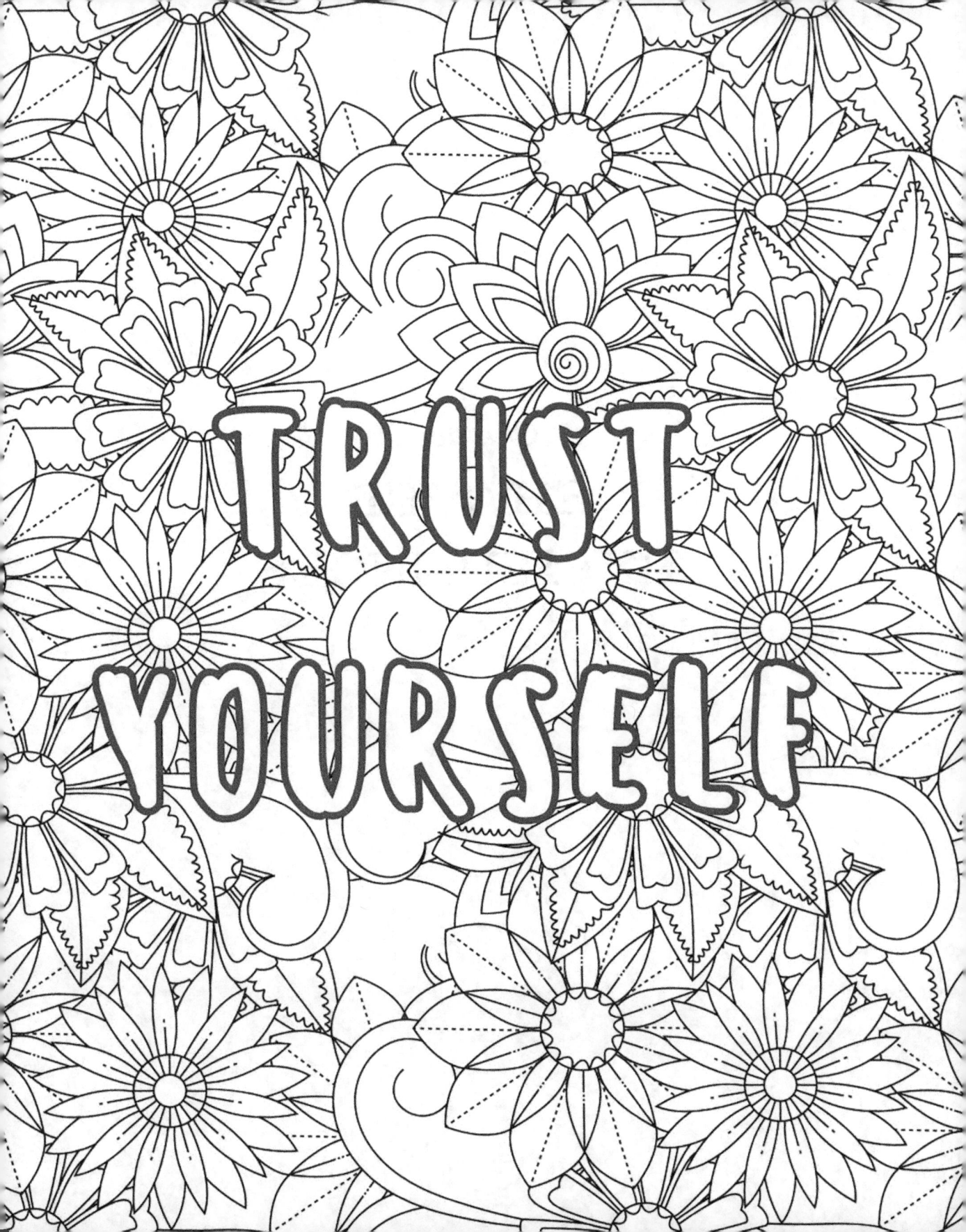

Chapter 2
SHAPED
EXPERIENCES

As you complete each exercise in this chapter,
you are making a commitment to live a life of
self-acceptance and unconditional self-love.
Each exercise will lead you on the path of
finding out which life experiences have shaped you.
Through this exploration, you will learn
who you really are and how to accept each part of you.
Through your brave acts of openness and
honesty with yourself, you liberate yourself
from living behind the mask.

What experiences shaped you into the person you are today?

These events can be positive or negative. They can come from your childhood or your recent past.

What happened to you? Who did it involve? How old were you?

This exercise requires you to think back on those life-shaping experiences. It is important that you reflect on the origin of what happened or what was said to understand the things that attribute to the way you think today. What lessons have stayed with you? Self-awareness occurs when you understand how these experiences have shaped you.

_____

_____

_____

_____

_____

_____

_____

_____

_____

_____

_____

_____

_____

_____

_____

_____

_____

_____

_____

_____

_____

_____

_____

_____

_____

_____

Liberation is Coming!!!

Be honest about how you view yourself. Do you know yourself? If you had to describe who you are, what would you say? What are your characteristics and personality traits? What makes you unique? What are your likes and dislikes? How do you view yourself?

Sometimes it can be challenging for people to speak about themselves with high regard whether they were taught to be modest, don't want people to view them as being arrogant, are not confident in how they see themselves, or worry about what others think of them, etc. It is my hope and desire that as you complete the exercises in this self-discovery workbook that you will become clear on who you are, which will lead you to self-love and ultimately self-acceptance.

Do not worry if the words don't come easily. Don't overthink it.

Allow me to introduce myself. I am:

_____

_____

_____

_____

_____

_____

_____

In this exercise, you will be asked to list anything you do not like about yourself. I know you may be asking, why? The answer is when you are aware and open to acknowledging flaws or traits that you are not pleased with, you are more open to accepting and working on it. This allows you to authentically show up without the mask, accepting and loving all of yourself unconditionally.

List anything you don't like about yourself and why.

_____

_____

_____

_____

_____

_____

List five things you like about yourself and why.

_____

_____

_____

_____

_____

_____

_____

Did you identify anything you do not like about yourself? If so, ask yourself if what you do not like can be changed. And if the answer is, "yes", are you willing to do what is required? These six steps provide a framework for transforming the dislikes into likes.

Remember during your journey to think positive thoughts, because your thoughts will impact your emotions.

Six Steps for Change

These six steps provide a framework for transforming the dislikes into likes.

1. Identify what you are not pleased with about yourself.

2. Determine if it is in your control to change.

3. If you control the ability to change, are you willing to do the work?

4. Apply your abilities and make a plan for the changes you want to see.

5. Give yourself grace, accept the person you are, and love yourself throughout the process.

6. Remember, what you say to yourself about yourself matters.

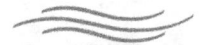

_____

_____

_____

_____

_____

_____

_____

_____

_____

_____

_____

_____

_____

_____

_____

_____

How Would You Define Your Communication Style?

	What does it mean?	Common characteristics	Verbal style	Non-verbal	Potential consequences
Passive	You put the rights of own. You minimize your self-worth.	You feel unimportant or like your feelings don't matter.	Speaks in a soft tone. Overly apologetic.	Doesn't maintain eye contact. Looks down or away.	Lowered self-esteem. Often disrespected. False feelings of inferiority.
Assertive	You stand up for your rights and respect the rights of others.	You believe in equality. We are all important.	Speaks in a firm tone. Takes ownership.	Maintains eye contact and a strong, positive posture.	Higher self-esteem and self-respect. Respected by others.
Aggressive	You stand up for your rights but violate the rights of others.	You believe you are superior. Only you are important.	Speaks in a loud tone. Places ownership elsewhere.	Intense eye contact. Clenched fists, finger points, and has a rigid posture.	Lowered self-esteem. Disrespect, fear and anger expressed by others.

_____

_____

_____

_____

_____

_____

How well do you communicate?

Do you address concerns that you have with family, friends, and peers?

Are you able to express your feelings?

Do you avoid conflict? Delay decision-making?

In this exercise, you will explore why you communicate the way that you do. Think back to three conversations you've had with a family member, a friend, and a peer. For each example, reflect on how you expressed yourself. Why did you say what you said? How did you say it? Do you wish you had said something differently? What prevented you from expressing honest feelings?

Explore how you respond to others.

_____

_____

_____

_____

_____

_____

_____

_____

_____

_____

_____

_____

_____

_____

_____

_____

_____

_____

_____

_____

_____

_____

_____

_____

_____

_____

Communication

Is your communication style beneficial in your relationships? Why do you choose to speak the way that you do? Identify the strengths in your communication style and opportunities for enhancing how you speak to others.

_____

_____

_____

_____

_____

_____

_____

_____

_____

_____

_____

_____

_____

What Makes You Happy?

Often, people get stuck answering the question, "What makes you happy?" When I ask clients, they often feel overwhelmed finding a suitable answer. The most common reason for this feeling is that they are lost in the titles they've gained and have forgotten who they are and what makes them happy. Also, some people overthink the question because they think there is only one correct answer. When it really is simple, as it relates to you. After much reflection, their usual response is, "I don't know."

You are the only one who can know. Happiness comes from within, and it is important that you know what makes you happy. Feeling centered and at peace is beneficial for your mental and physical wellbeing. On this self-discovery journey, explore what brings you happiness, peace, and contentment. Here are some examples of activities that can be helpful.

- Spending time reading a book or magazine that you enjoy
- A walk in the park
- A favorite meal or TV show
- Traveling and exploring new spaces
- Spending time with family and friends

So, I will ask again. What makes you happy?

_____

_____

_____

_____

_____

When do you feel at peace?

_____

_____

_____

_____

_____

When are you content?

_____

_____

_____

_____

_____

Do you listen to your body, and know when to take a break?

_____

_____

_____

_____

_____

Are you pouring from an empty cup, and if yes, why?

_____

_____

_____

_____

What boundaries have you establish to take care of you?

_____

_____

_____

_____

What is your self-care regimen?

_____

_____

_____

_____

_____

_____

_____

_____

_____

_____

_____

_____

_____

_____

_____

_____

_____

_____

_____

_____

_____

_____

_____

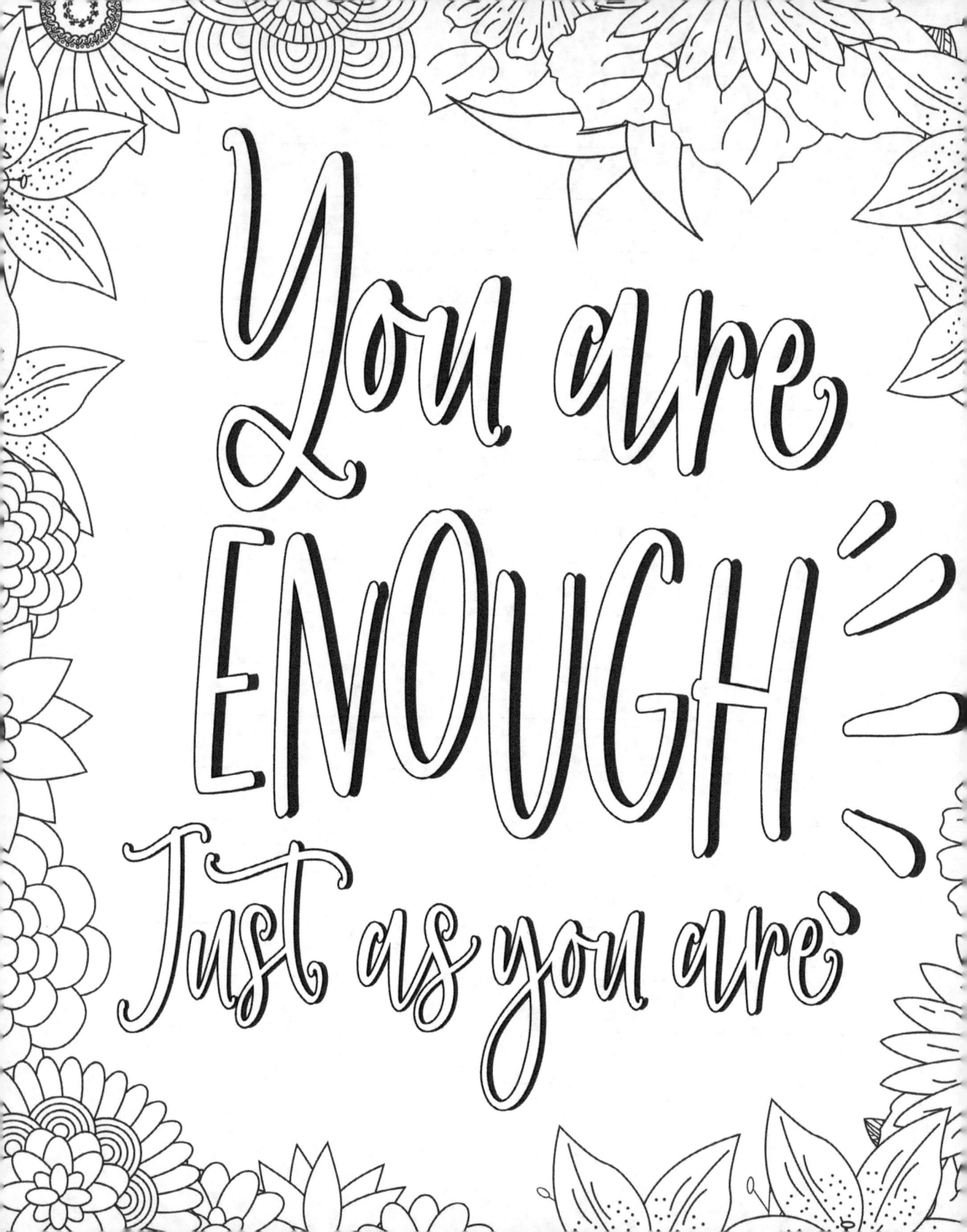

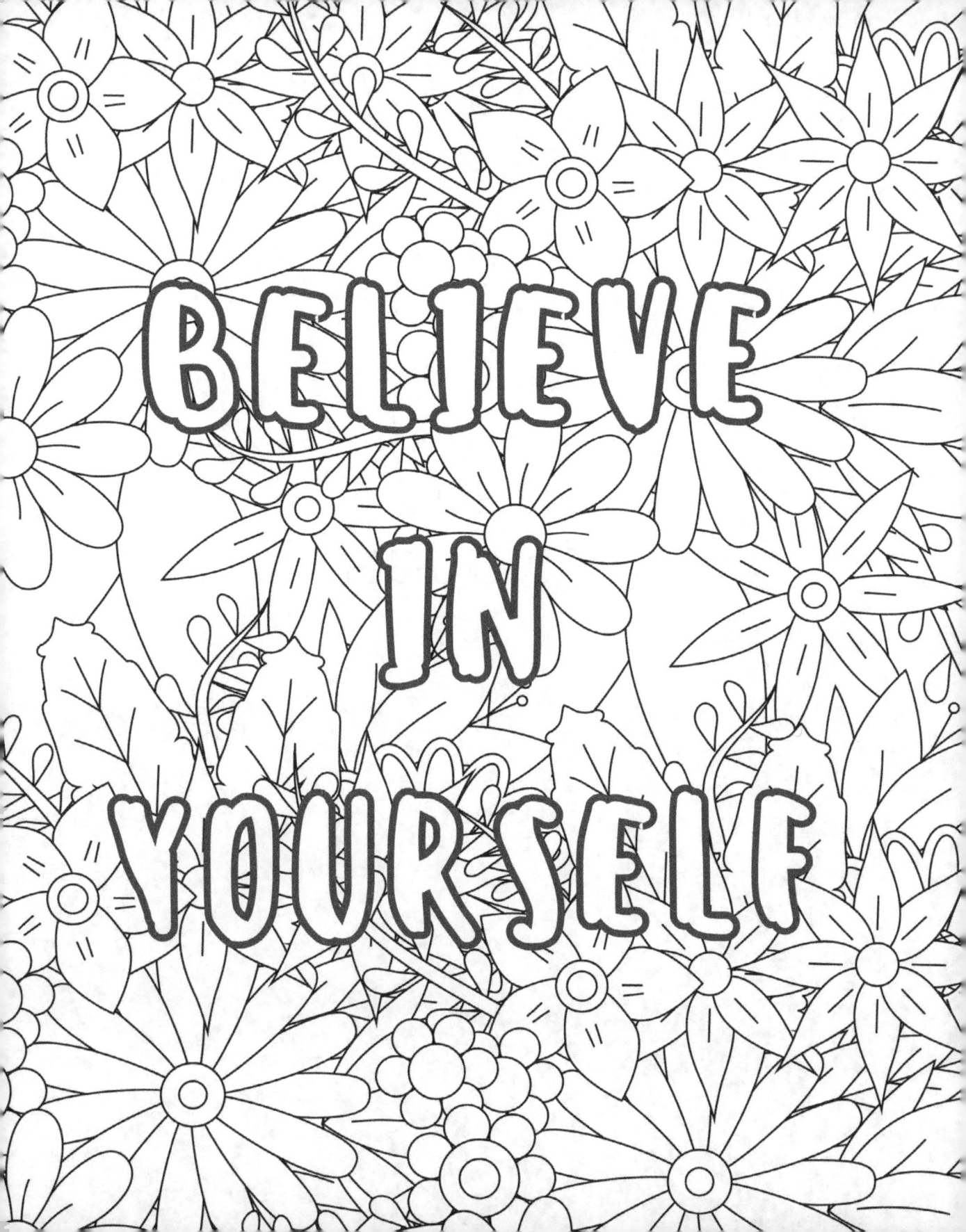

Chapter 3

I AM
ENOUGH

Do you seek validation from others?

First, let me say, there is nothing wrong with wanting recognition or validation. As children, receiving validation for our efforts help build self-esteem and confidence. Reassurance from parents, teachers, family, and friends is valuable when you experience early successes and failures. As we get older, it is acceptable to ask opinions of others and to want recognition for achieving personal and professional goals.

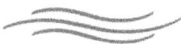

You should be self-aware of when and why you are seeking validation from others. Sometimes the validation that you seek from others is because you haven't received it and now long for validation. When validation hasn't been received, a person can feel unworthy or unsure of themselves, which can lead them to seek validation from others. Also, desiring others to tell them that they are enough and that they can achieve the goal(s). The danger in that is, if you don't receive the validation, you can start to question your abilities, and it can lead to you being stuck. Validating yourself is an important part of building self-esteem and confidence.

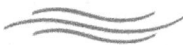

Self-validation is crucial to a healthy self-esteem. If you are putting the opinions, approval, and recognition of others over your own, you will likely often seek that external validation. This can lead to not feeling good enough, self-doubt, indecisiveness, anxiety, depression, low self-esteem, and the list goes on... Moving forward, take the pledge, validate yourself!

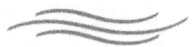

In this exercise, reflect on the times in your life when you sought validation. In your replies, try answering these questions:

How are these events still impacting you today?

Why were you seeking the validation?

What could someone else give you that you could not give yourself?

_____

_____

_____

_____

_____

_____

_____

_____

_____

_____

_____

Positive Traits

Take a few moments to identify all the positive traits you possess. Whenever you doubt your abilities, review these traits and acknowledge all the wonderful parts of you. Remember, you are not limited to the items on this list.

Dependable	Humorous	Loveable	Teachable	Smart
Kind	Energetic	Friendly	Strong	Accepting
Optimistic	Respectable	Reliable	Self-Directed	Creative
Honest	Patient	Resilient	Loyal	Caring
Skilled	Open Minded	Confident	Brave	Decisive
Grateful	Positive	Innovative	Realistic	Generous
Nurturing	Hardworking	Focused	Independent	Humble
Forgiving	Adaptable	Committed	Fair	Determined
Dedicated	Flexible	Organized	Sincere	Courageous
Persevering	Appreciative	Polite	Trustworthy	Adventurous
Selfless	Knowledgeable	Efficient	Sociable	Self-Reliant
Ambitious	Empathetic	Natural-leader	Self-Disciplined	Assertive

In this exercise, select three to five of your positive traits. Reflect on how these traits help you and others. Explain how the trait positively impacts your life and your relationships.

_____

_____

_____

_____

_____

_____

_____

_____

_____

_____

_____

_____

_____

_____

_____

_____

_____

_____

_____

_____

_____

_____

_____

_____

_____

_____

_____

_____

_____

_____

_____

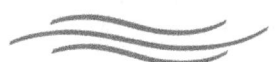

*See yourself beyond
the traits you listed.
See yourself beyond
what has held you
back in the past.
You have everything
within you to achieve
anything you desire.
You are already enough.*

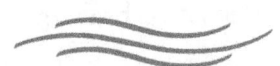

Do you have the need to please?

This is an important question to ask yourself because as you are discovering who you are, you need to be self-aware. Are you making choices and saying yes to people because you want to present yourself as a nice, helpful, always there if someone needs you, never say no person because you think not doing so means rejection or that you are being a mean person? Are you wanting people to like you, so you say yes, even when you don't want to?

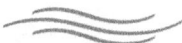

There are so many reasons why people have the need to please, but know that the most common reason is seeking acceptance and wanting to be included, liked or loved. Unfortunately, the harsh truth is that you can say yes or do what everyone asks of you, and still not be accepted, liked or loved. This is sometimes challenging for people to hear, because as humans we all desire to be wanted, liked and loved, but it is important that we live in reality knowing that everyone will not like you no matter how kind you may be or think you are.

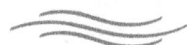

Also, the need to please can make you an enabler, which hinders people's growth. Oftentimes we don't discuss what the need to please syndrome gives the person that always says yes. But sometimes there is a reward for them, too: the rescuer or savior feeling, praise for helping, ability to boast or brag, etc.

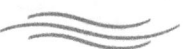

It is important that when you are making choices and doing for others that you ask yourself this one crucial question. What is my intent? Why am I doing this or saying yes to? When you are clear on your intent and it serves you in a good way then move forward. If you are doing it for the need to please ask yourself: How am I showing up authentic and genuine? Why am I desiring to please someone else at the cost of my integrity for myself (not being authentic and genuine to yourself is you not being honest to yourself)? You can't expect others to have integrity and honesty to you when you can't be that for yourself.... Period!

Do you look to please others? If so, who do you consistently aim to please and why? How is this behavior serving you? If this behavior negatively impacts you, forgive yourself and make strides to improve your behavior.

_____

_____

_____

_____

_____

_____

_____

Did you ever have the need to please? If yes, acknowledge it and forgive yourself for anything that you may still be holding on to.

_____

_____

_____

_____

_____

_____

_____

_____

_____

_____

_____

_____

_____

_____

_____

_____

_____

_____

_____

_____

_____

_____

_____

_____

_____

Positive Traits

```
F G A F B A I O R G A N I Z E D X M K V K U N R
O E R U B A N O L U F E T A R G N N A X W V R R
C S Q N W D D V U H O G X C O U R T E O U S W B
U C F N E J E Y R A T V C O N F I D E N T I B I
S D B Y V S P C L R R Y M O T I V A T E D V V G
E E I K I U E W Z U W N L F U H G U O H T B N S
D D N W T O N V L E V N D L S I K S B W V Z Z X
D N N Y I R D L S O Y E D R E S P E C T A B L E
J I O N S E E O R R N C I E F P X P Q W C I D T
F M V L O N N G T K Y Q O R T U L B G X J N G N
T N A K P E T N U I Z K Y P F C R O R Y I O N E
Z E T M M G E C G N I B P U T A E F Y K S T O I
Z P I J I L E D O G L P N R V I O R P A R S R T
S O V L I R Q K E M B Y H E X E M E I H L U T A
S J E S U N E E T T P B Q C E R J I B D E F S P
G E E E P V T A V G E A I T C U G Q S X F P B N
N R N D L E E E L I N R S J G T N H T T K L I K
J Q J S E B J L L I T I M S M A S S E F I V E D
L Q B O I C I U B L S C R I I M N E M L O C S S
D Q V J S T I X R A I T A U N O U J N A P A N J
W U Y L K R I Y E I S I G N T E N Q J O R F L X
G Q S Y U C P V I L C L E C T R D A P T U T U F
L W A H E H D C E V F N E N X T U U T H B H C L
```

self-directed helpful patient mature decisive independent
realistic skilled determined optimistic compassionate sensitive
nurturing open-minded innovative brave generous motivated
grateful courteous organized focused positive resilient intelligent
reliable respectable honest confident thoughtful flexible kind
friendly strong creative funny attractive loyal hardworking smart

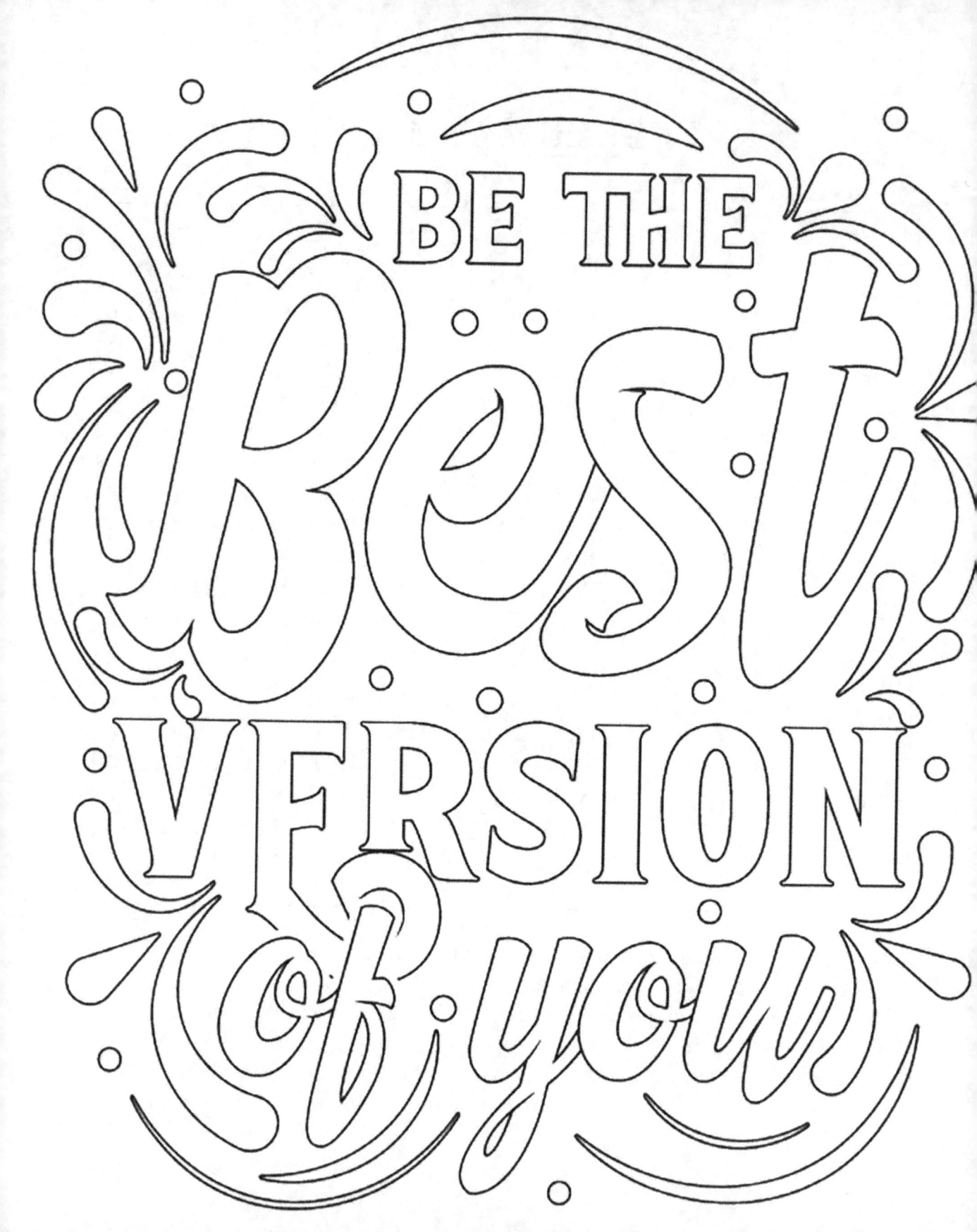

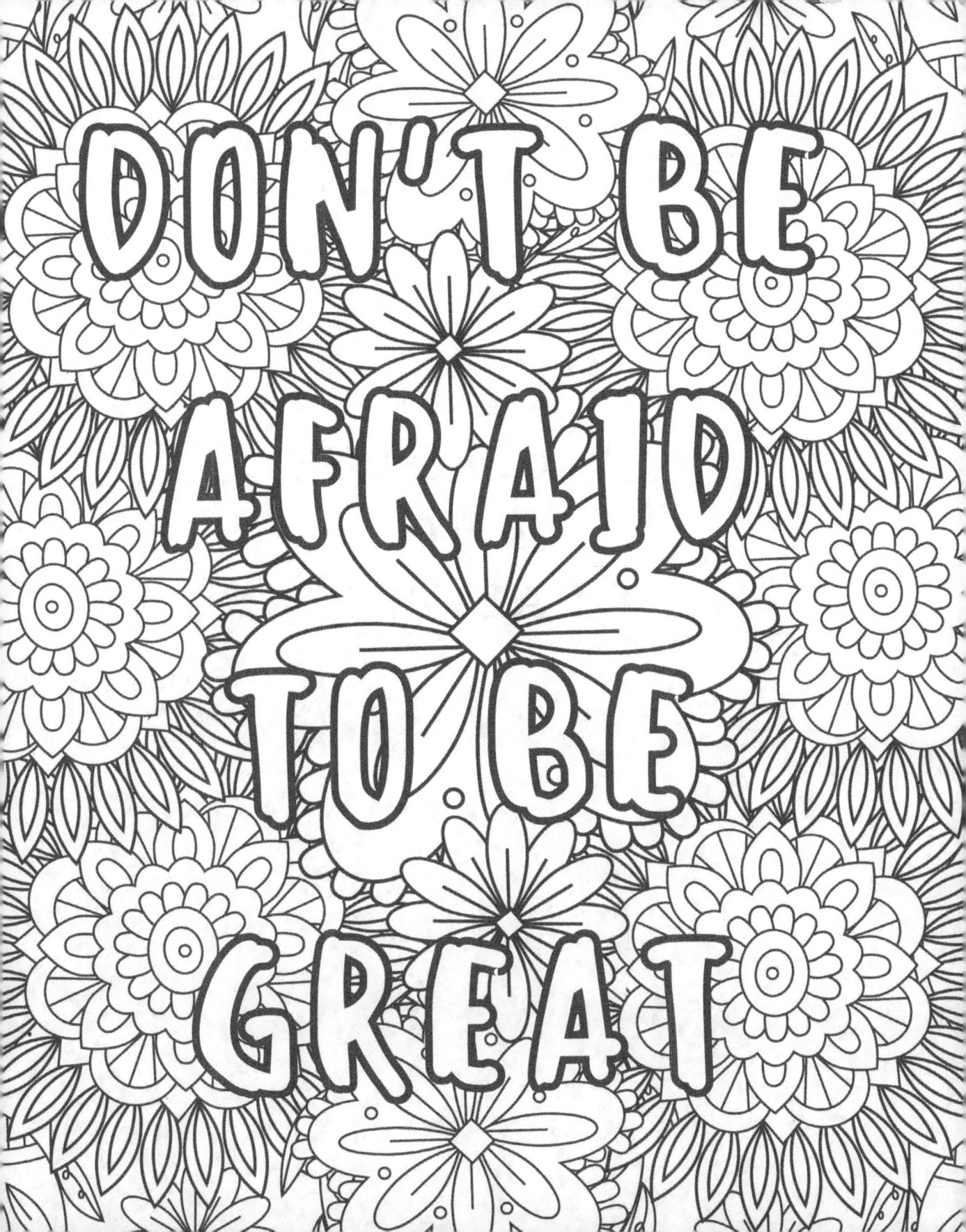

Chapter 4

STRENGTHS
AND
QUALITIES

How well do I know myself?

Knowing who you are, what you value, and who you want to become will develop your confidence. In this exercise, reflect on your accomplishments. Recognize your strengths, qualities, and abilities.

What do I value most?

_____

_____

_____

_____

What am I good at?

_____

_____

_____

_____

What talents do I possess?

_____

_____

_____

_____

What things make me unique?

_____

_____

_____

_____

What challenges have I overcome?

_____

_____

_____

_____

What are my goals?

_____

_____

_____

_____

Continue to explore your qualities. Read each trait and share about a time where you represented its meaning. How did you display the trait? How did it make you feel?

Kind

_____

_____

_____

_____

_____

Selfless

_____

_____

_____

_____

_____

Sacrifice

_____

_____

_____

_____

_____

Courageous

_____

_____

_____

_____

_____

Loving

_____

_____

_____

_____

_____

Determined

_____

_____

_____

_____

_____

Happiness

_____

_____

_____

_____

_____

Affirming Yourself

Creating I AM statements is a very positive exercise. If you are struggling or feel unaccomplished you can often turn your feelings around with a review of some positive I AM statements.

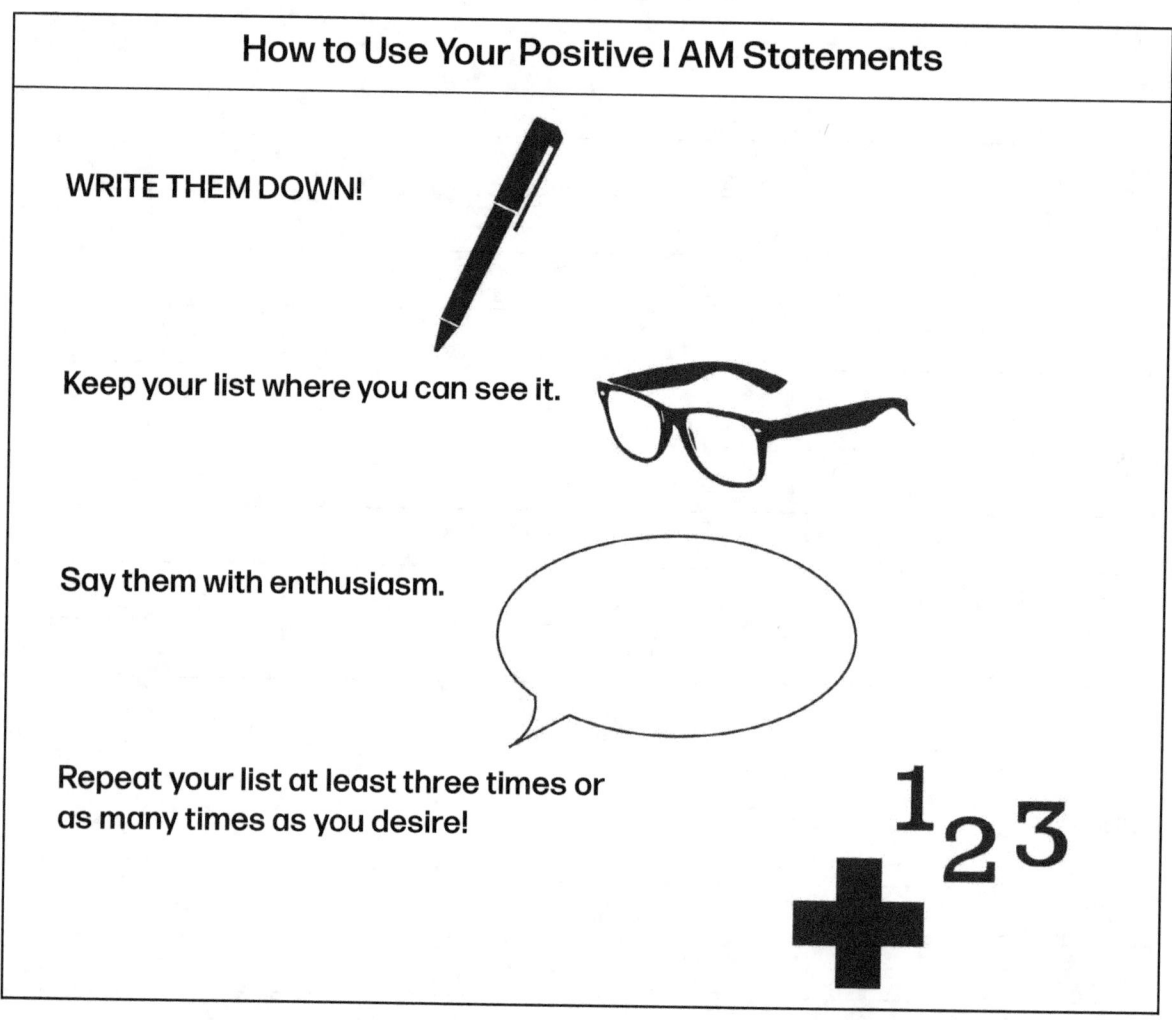

How to Use Your Positive I AM Statements

WRITE THEM DOWN!

Keep your list where you can see it.

Say them with enthusiasm.

Repeat your list at least three times or as many times as you desire!

Create your positive I Am statements

1. *I am capable of achieving any goal I commit to.*
2. _____
3. _____
4. _____
5. _____
6. _____
7. _____
8. _____
9. _____
10. _____
11. _____
12. _____
13. _____
14. _____
15. _____
16. _____
17. _____
18. _____
19. _____
20. _____

Strength in Knowing Your Weaknesses

For some people, it is difficult to admit their personal weakness. Oftentimes, we focus on our strengths because they make us feel good. Exploring your weaknesses is essential. Your weaknesses allow you to build your own path for development. Understanding where you can improve will expand your confidence. Once you realize there is strength, even in weakness, you will embrace yourself, flaws and all.

Write your weaknesses in the circle. Acknowledge each one by reading them aloud. Process any thoughts or emotions that come up. In the space below the circle, plan for improvement. Write the actions you will take to resolve the weaknesses that negatively impact your life.

_____

_____

_____

_____

_____

_____

_____

_____

_____

_____

_____

_____

_____

_____

_____

_____

_____

_____

_____

Accomplishment Exercise

What life experiences are you proud of?

Often through school, work, church, sports, and community activities we are able to display our gifts and talents. Write four of your accomplishments. Consider the strengths and qualities you used or developed to achieve the goal.

Accomplishments	Skills, Strengths, and Qualities

_____

_____

_____

_____

_____

_____

_____

_____

_____

_____

_____

_____

_____

_____

_____

_____

_____

_____

_____

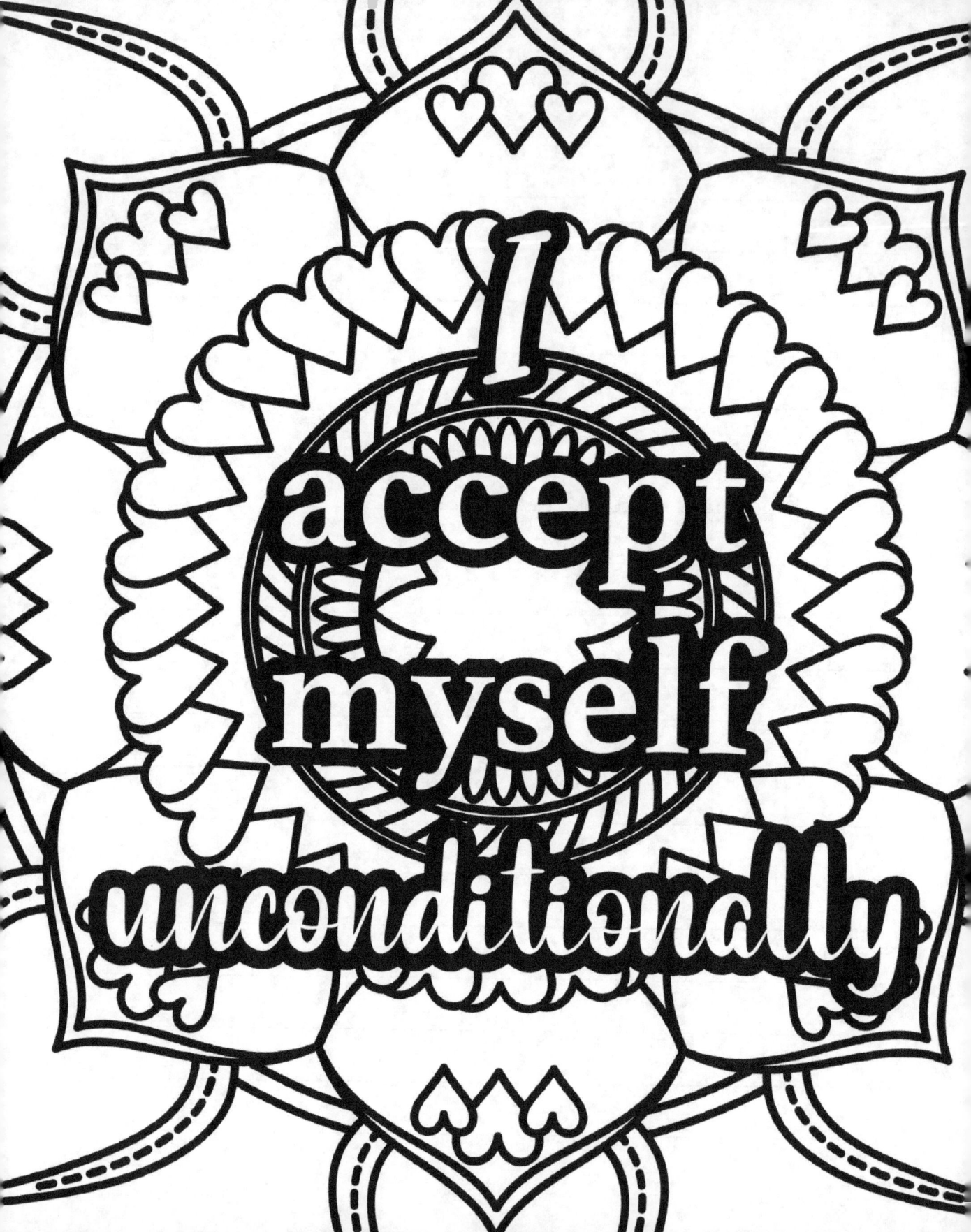

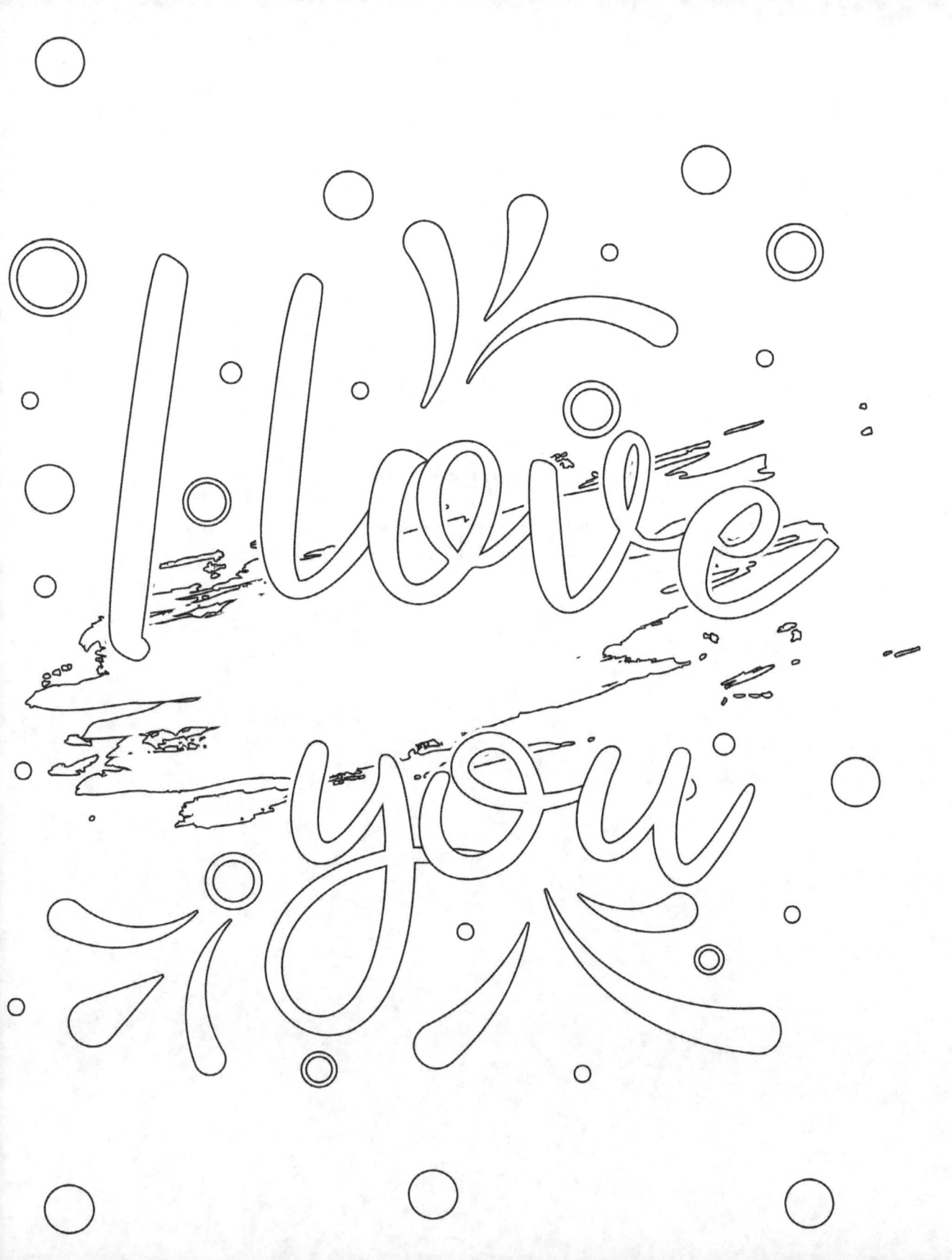

Chapter 5

SELF-ACCEPTANCE

What does it mean to have self-acceptance?

Self-acceptance means unconditionally accepting all parts of you. Accept your weaknesses and strengths and positive and negative imperfections of yourself. It is complete acceptance of oneself.

Key Practices to Achieve Self-Acceptance

- Accept All of You
- Have Compassion for Yourself
- Embracing Who You Are
- Accepting Your Personality, Physical Attributes, Skills and Abilities
- Accept Your Strengths and Weaknesses
- Do Not Harshly Judge Yourself

Benefits of practicing Self-Acceptance

- High Self-Acceptance Leads To Better Mood Regulation
- Liberation To Be Yourself
- More Open To Take Risk With Less Worry Or Fear
- Living Authentically
- Improved Self- Esteem
- Autonomy Over Your Own Life

The exercises you complete throughout this workbook will guide you through a path of self-discovery. You can achieve self-acceptance when you are aware of all the parts of you. When you can identify what makes you unique, you can see how special you are. This exploration reveals the areas in which you are strong and opportunities for you to improve the pieces of you that will help you thrive throughout your life.

Six-Step Exercise to bring you further into your quest to Self-Acceptance.

Forgiveness Exercise

Step 1. Forgiveness: Showing compassion to yourself. If you are holding on to past mistakes and regrets, forgive yourself for the decisions. Learn from the experiences and release it. Start living in the present (today)because you cannot change the past. Staying in the past (reminiscing) on what you should have done will keep you stuck. Release it and move forward. During this exercise, journal the things that you need to forgive yourself for.

_____

_____

_____

_____

_____

_____

_____

_____

_____

_____

_____

My Thoughts About Me

Step 2. Identify the thoughts that make you not want to accept you. In this exercise, journal your thoughts of feeling ashamed, guilty, unworthy, and not enough. When completing this exercise, don't judge yourself, but make yourself aware of the parts you are not accepting of.

What steps do you need to take to accept those parts?

_____

_____

_____

_____

_____

_____

_____

_____

_____

_____

_____

_____

_____

_____

_____

_____

_____

_____

_____

_____

_____

_____

_____

_____

_____

_____

_____

_____

_____

_____

_____

Exploring Feelings

Step 3. Explore the feelings and emotions that come from your thoughts and experiences. Be kind to all of your emotions. Use this time to discover how you process your feelings. Show yourself compassion as you would to someone you care about.

_____

_____

_____

_____

_____

_____

_____

_____

_____

_____

_____

_____

_____

How Perfection has Impacted Me?

Step 4. Embrace not being perfect: Accepting your imperfections is crucial to self-acceptance. Knowing that no one, including yourself, is perfect, and everyone, including yourself, will make mistakes. It is good to view all your success and failures as experiences and not allow either to define who you are. In this exercise, journal how wanting to be perfect has impacted you. Did it have you putting off completing tasks, anxious and worried, afraid you or your actions weren't good enough, etc.?

_____

_____

_____

_____

_____

_____

_____

_____

_____

_____

_____

Authentically Me

Step 5. Stay in your lane: Don't look to the right or the left of you to compare yourself with others. When you compare yourself to others you will be challenged with accepting yourself. You were created to be authentically you. In this exercise, journal about all parts of who you are.

_____

_____

_____

_____

_____

_____

_____

_____

_____

_____

_____

_____

_____

How Does My Inner Circle Make Me Feel?

Step 6. In this exercise express how your friend group makes you feel. Work on creating an accepting inner circle by surrounding yourself with people who support and embrace you for who you are. Show the same acceptance to others. In this exercise, journal ways you can meet or connect with people that are accepting of people being authentically themselves.

_____

_____

_____

_____

_____

_____

_____

_____

_____

_____

_____

_____

_____

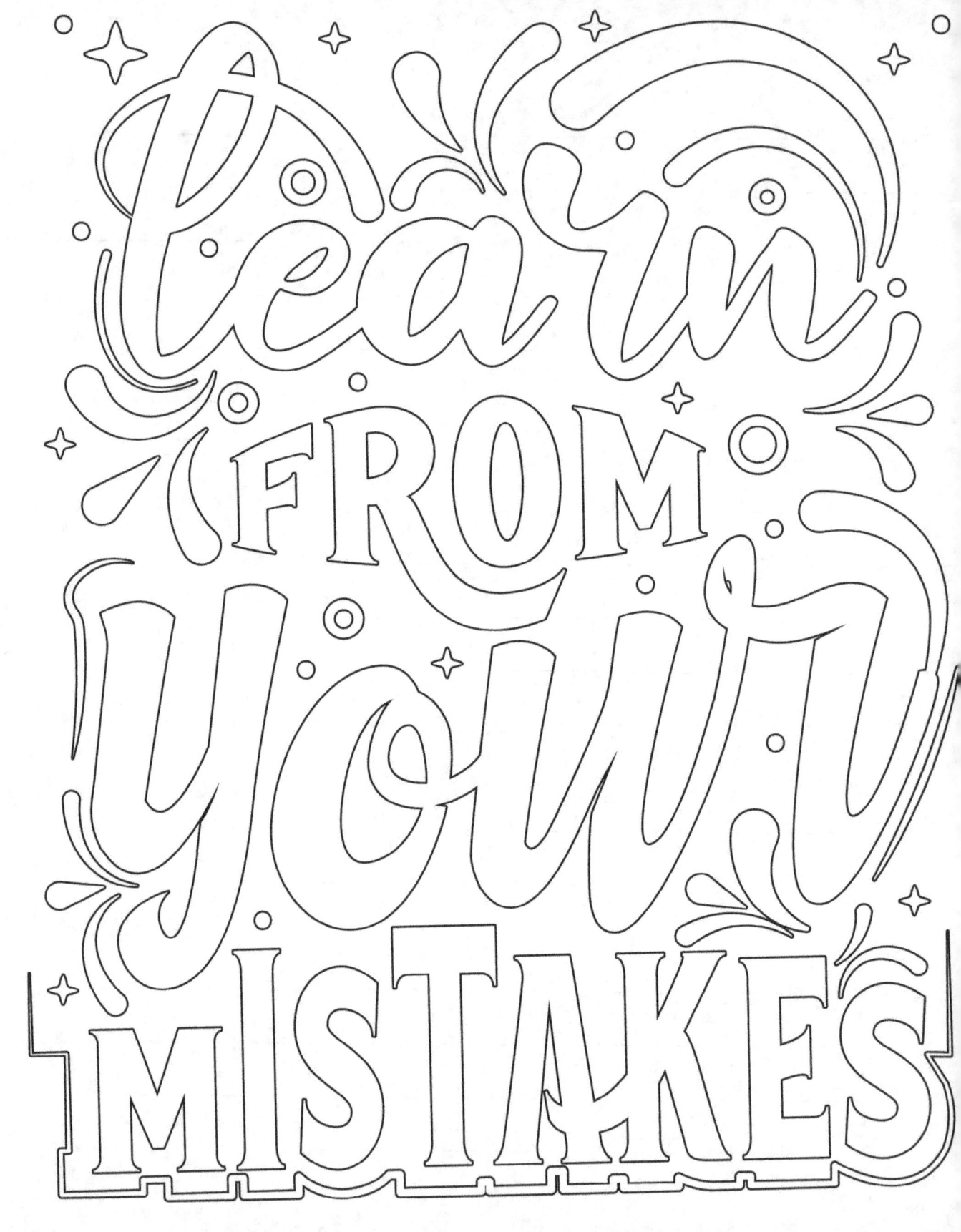

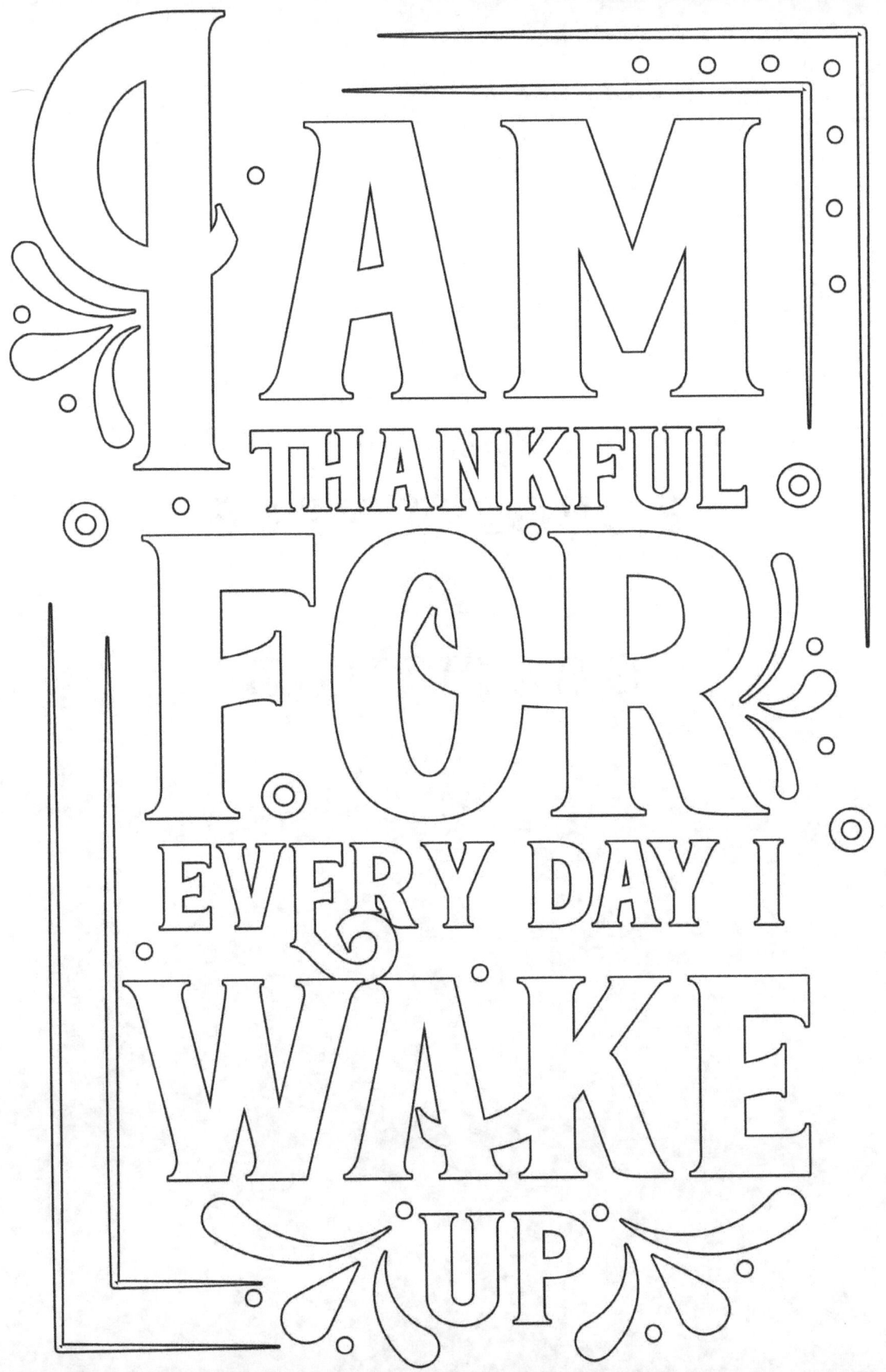

Chapter 6

FORGIVENESS
AND
GRATITUDE

Self-forgiveness Can Liberate and Empower!!!

The inability to move past guilt and self-doubt may take a toll on our daily lives. Particularly, struggling to forgive ourselves for our actions can be damaging to self-esteem; the more we suffer, the greater the potential impact on our productivity, mood, and state of mind.

Time to Heal

Define what you would like to forgive yourself for

- Identify the negative emotions you will release

- Acknowledge the benefits of self-forgiveness: for yourself and for others

- Make a dedicated commitment to forgive yourself

The capacity to forgive ourselves for mistakes is essential to our well-being. Deciding to let go and process feelings can be difficult and may take time to move through the process, but the benefits are unlimited. In the upcoming exercises, work through your self-forgiveness at your own pace.

Do you need to forgive yourself? If so, what for? You can start by writing, "I want to forgive myself for".

_____

_____

_____

_____

_____

_____

Acknowledge any negative emotions that you want to release. Is there anything preventing you from having inner peace and joy? Example: criticisms, blame, guilt, anger, regret, frustration, and unhappiness. Use this space to write and release.

_____

_____

_____

_____

_____

_____

_____

Acknowledge the benefits of self-forgiveness. Describe the advantages of freeing yourself from these negative emotions. The benefits may be short or long-term. The possibilities include increased trust, a clear conscious, and a renewed focus on what makes you happy. Start your work in the space provided to plan for your own forgiveness.

_____

_____

_____

_____

_____

Consider how forgiving yourself will benefit others. Acknowledge how forgiving yourself will benefit others. Consider how your self-forgiveness might be valuable to those around you or the person you have wronged. Example: "I will be a more patient person." Some of these benefits might relate to your answers directly above.

_____

_____

_____

_____

_____

_____

Commit to the process of self-forgiveness. Using your answers to the previous question, create a commitment pledge: "I commit to forgiving myself for _____ and open myself to the benefit of _____."

_____

_____

_____

_____

_____

_____

_____

_____

_____

_____

_____

_____

_____

_____

Is there anything holding you back?

Examine your thoughts, emotions, and relationships. Are they holding you back? It may be something that was said or thoughts you had about yourself that you cannot let go of. Describe these events and any negative emotions associated.

_____

_____

_____

_____

_____

_____

_____

_____

_____

_____

_____

_____

_____

Acknowledging Mistakes and Taking Responsibility of the Consequences.

Accepting positive feedback or recognition is easy, but there are times when we all have made mistakes. It is important to understand that our actions can have negative consequences to ourself or others. When this occurs, we must accept our actions and learn from our mistake through acknowledging, taking accountability, having remorse, apologizing to anyone that you hurt and to yourself in hopes to make a mend with others and forgive yourself.

_____

_____

_____

_____

_____

_____

_____

_____

_____

_____

_____

_____

What are you thankful for?

An Attitude of Gratitude

Gratitude is an emotion like appreciation, and positive psychological research has found neurological reasons why so many people can benefit from this general practice of expressing thanks for our lives, even in times of challenge and change.

The Harvard Medical School provides more detail, writing that gratitude is: "A thankful appreciation for what an individual receives, whether tangible or intangible. With gratitude, people acknowledge the goodness in their lives... As a result, gratitude also helps people connect to something larger than themselves as individuals–whether to other people, nature, or a higher power."

Benefits of Gratitude

- Better health; less physical and mental fatigue

- Developed patience, humility, and wisdom

- Greater resiliency

- Increased satisfaction and positivity

(Positive Psychology.com)

Gratitude Exercise

Reflect on what you are grateful for in your life. Use this space to identify your gratitude for all the wonderful things in your life.

_____

_____

_____

_____

_____

_____

_____

_____

_____

_____

_____

_____

_____

_____

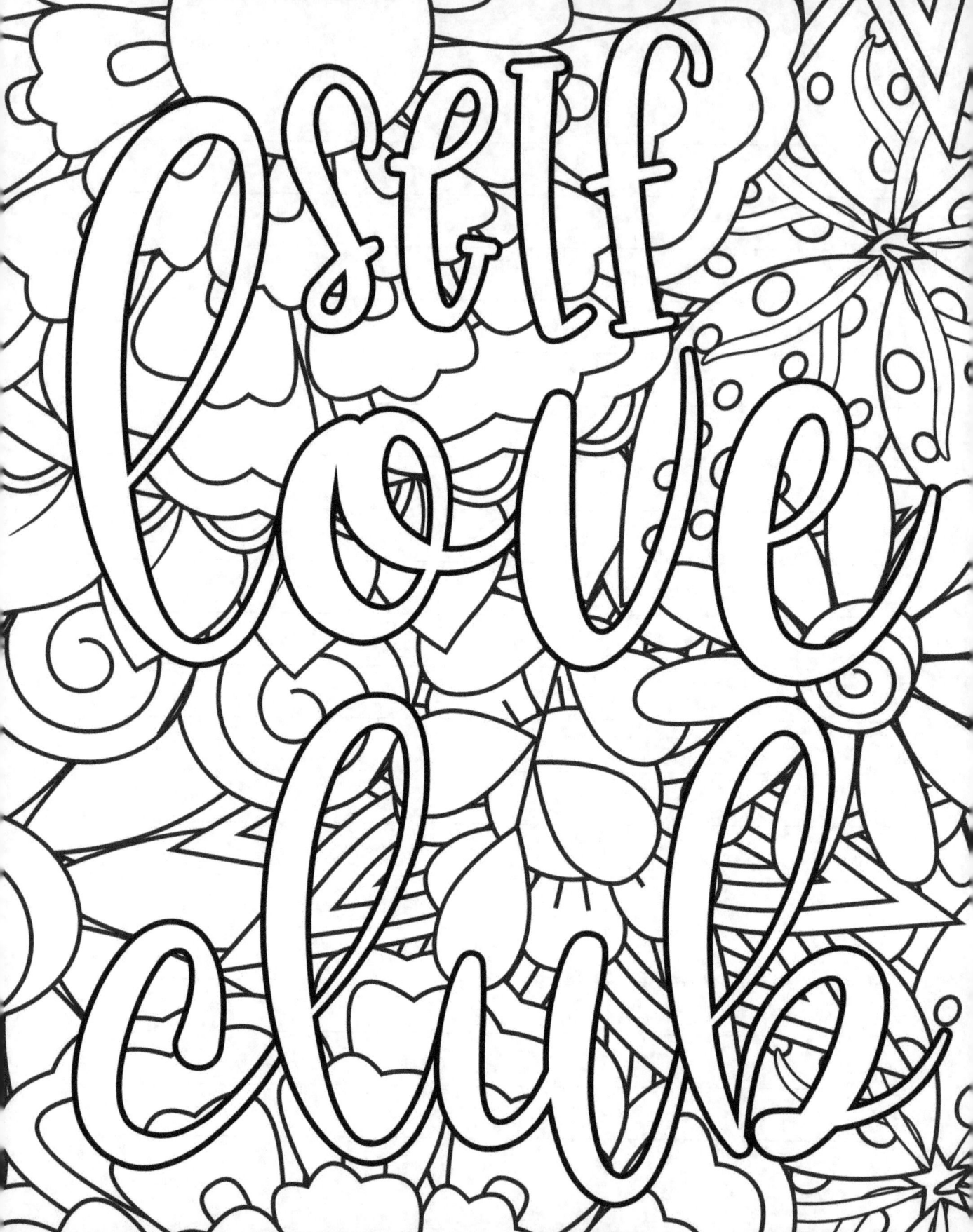

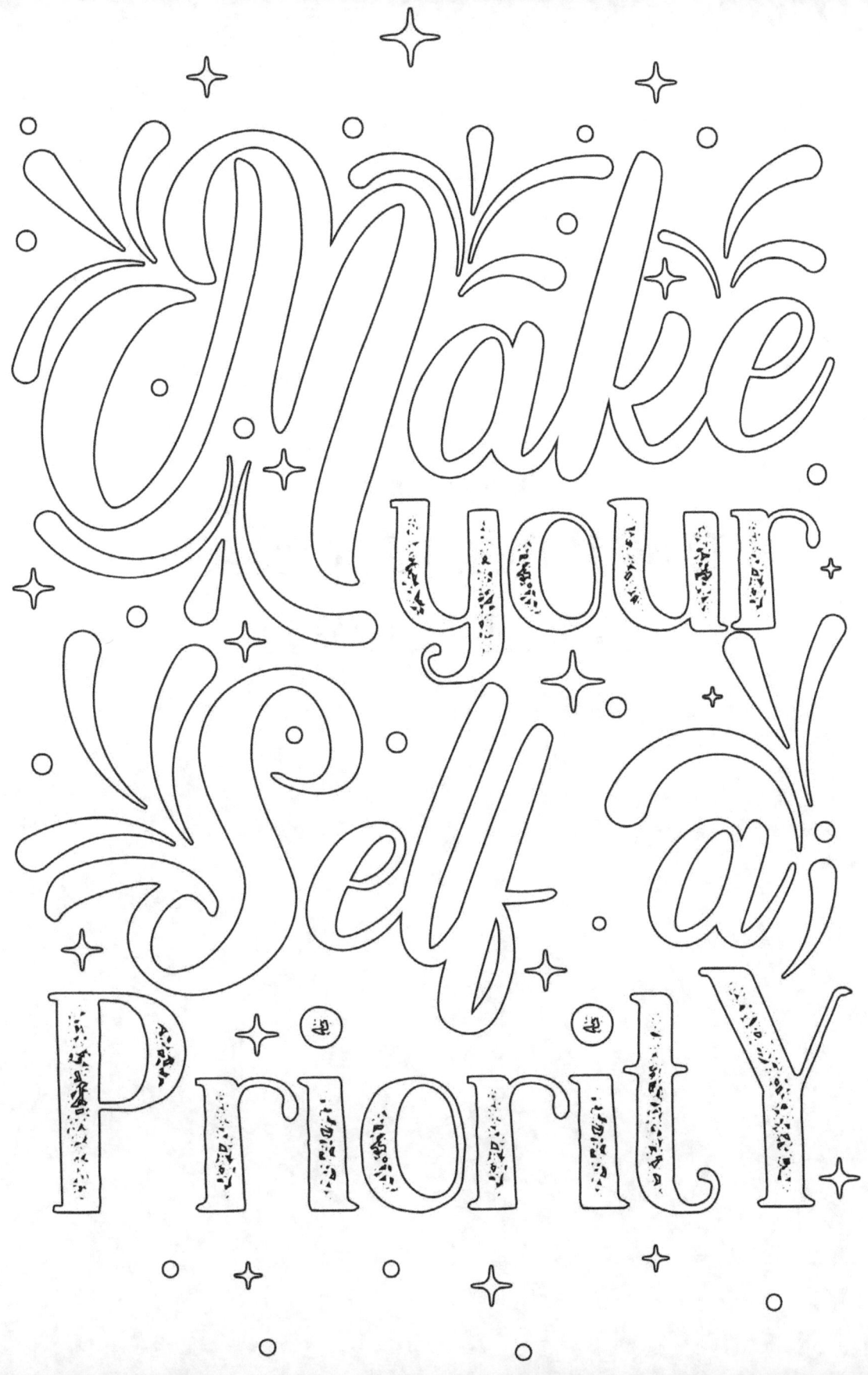

Chapter 7

UNCONDITIONAL
SELF-LOVE

Self-Love

Many people are unsure how to genuinely love themselves. Some people may not feel worthy of love. Others may not have received love or been taught how to love themselves. Do you know how to love yourself? In this exercise, explore the ways you can practice self-love.

How do you love yourself?

Show yourself respect, take care of yourself, be kind to you and responsible for you.

Self-respect:

Use your voice. Speak up when others hurt your feelings. Communicate your needs.
Know your worth. Create standards and values that you are not willing to compromise.

Self-compassion:

Be kind to you. Forgive your mistakes and imperfections.
Be your cheerleader. Use your positive affirmations to chase away doubt and fear.

Self-care:

Find your happy. Explore the things that bring you joy and do more of them.
Make yourself a priority. Meet your needs before caring for others.
Total well-being. Make time to care for your mind, body, and soul.
Make peace with your past. Do the work to heal from the past and embrace your future.

What does it mean to love yourself unconditionally?

Accept your weaknesses and your strengths. Explore all the wonderful things that make you, you. Unconditional love means choosing to love everything you find on the journey of you.

How do you achieve unconditional self-love?

Unconditional self-love is achieved through self-acceptance, which is an important part of developing healthy relationships with others. Loving yourself means recognizing your own self-worth and living your own life as honestly as you can, being authentically you.

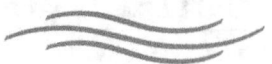

- Start with self-respect (value yourself enough to create standards and values that you are not willing to compromise).

- Accept your strengths and weaknesses unapologetically. Being authentic, vulnerable, and carefree regardless of other opinions.

- Do not compare yourself to others.

- Be truly honest with yourself (show up authentically you.) Forgive yourself for mistakes and imperfections.

- Remind yourself of your positive qualities each day. By using positive affirmations, you will feel better about yourself and your ability to take on the day.

- Make yourself a priority. Prioritize your health and happiness. Often, people are so busy caring for others that they put their own needs to the side. Don't do this. You are of no value to anyone else if you are sick or unhappy; you cannot pour from an empty cup.

- Make your needs clear. If someone in your life is letting you down, make sure they are fully aware of what you need.

- Nurture yourself. Think of what brings you peace and do more of it.

- Make peace with your past. Do the work to heal so you can let go of old hurts and allow yourself to move forward to embrace the present.

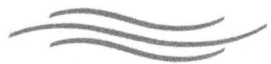

What does self-care mean to you?

How do you feel about self-care?

_____

_____

_____

How much personal time do you need to feel rejuvenated?

_____

_____

_____

How would you use more self-care time?

_____

_____

_____

Are your personal needs being met?

_____

_____

_____

What makes you feel calm and at peace?

_____

_____

_____

Suggested Self-Care Exercises

- Find a comfortable space to relax or catch-up on sleep

- Meditate

- Nature walks

- Yoga and exercise

- Read an enjoyable book

- Pamper yourself with a massage or spa day

- Make time to enjoy your favorite TV shows or movies

- Cook or try a new recipe for enjoyment

- Take a trip to a new place or visit friends and family

- Explore new hobbies, like arts and crafts or other things that interest you

- Do what is relaxing, rejuvenating, and makes you happy

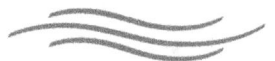

Self-Care Scrabble

1. IARALOTEXN _____

2. BATEHRNIG ESSCEEXRI _____

3. ITMEETDA _____

4. DEAR _____

5. WKAL _____

6. SPLEE _____

7. GAYO _____

8. REECEXIS _____

9. CIAZLSIEO _____

10. ATBHE _____

11. CLORO _____

12. MFNRAIFTSAIO _____

13. NETFEROICL _____

14. MCISU _____

15. UJRNLAO _____

16. SUMNMAETE TITYVAIC _____

17. CKOO _____

18. ASEMG _____

19. ELPUZZS _____

20. GDENARGNI _____

Awesome job!!

*I am excited that you've went on
your self-discovery journey. It
has made you recall your past,
be aware of your present, and figure
out your future. You are now able to
tell your narrative from your experiences
and through becoming self-aware. As you
complete this last exercise, it is imperative that
you, as the author, accept yourself authentically,
loving all parts of you unconditionally, so that you
can live a life of liberation moving forward!!*

My Past, Present, and Future

This is about who you were in the past, who you are today, and who you want to be in the future. Use this space to explore your unique story.

_____

_____

_____

_____

_____

_____

_____

_____

_____

_____

_____

_____

_____

_____

_____

_____

_____

_____

_____

_____

_____

_____

_____

_____

_____

_____

_____

_____

_____

_____

_____

_____

_____

_____

_____

_____

_____

_____

_____

_____

_____

_____

_____

_____

_____

_____

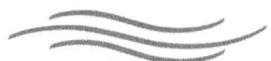

*I hope that this self-discovery workbook
was the start of your continuous work of
accepting and loving yourself unconditionally.
This workbook is not a replacement for
therapy, so I encourage you to seek
therapy if you have realized from your
self-discovery that you need healing
or support to continue accepting
and loving yourself unconditionally!!*

_____

_____

_____

_____

_____

_____

_____

_____

_____

_____

_____

_____

_____

_____

_____

_____

_____

_____

```
F   A F   I O R G A N I Z E D
O   U N   L U F E T A R G
C   N   D   H     C O U R T E O U S
U   N E   E Y   A   C O N F I D E N T
S D   Y V S P   L R   M O T I V A T E D
E E I   I U E     D   L U F T H G U O H T
D D N   T O N     W N D E L L I K S
  N N   I R D     O   E D R E S P E C T A B L E
  I O   S E E     R     I E             D T
  M V   O N N   T K   O R T   L B     N G N
  N A   P E T N   I     P F C R O     I   N E
  E T   G E C   N       T A E   Y K     O I
  P I   L   D O G   V I   R   P A   R     R T
  O V   I R   E M     E X   E M   I   L   T A
S E S   N E E   T P     R   I   D     S P
  E E E   T A V G E A     U     S   F
N R N D L   E E L I N R S     T N H   T T   L
    S E B   L L I T I M S A S S E   I   E
      I C I   B L S C R I I M   E M L   C   S
      T I X   A I T A U N O   N A P
W U Y L   I S E   I G I R T E N   O R F
G O S Y U C P V I L   E C T R D A   H T U
L W A H E   E V F N E N   T U U T     L
E V I T A E R C   E   R T   A N   E
```

self-directed   helpful   patient   mature   decisive   independent
realistic   skilled   determined   optimistic   compassionate   sensitive
nurturing   open-minded   innovative   brave   generous   motivated
grateful   courteous   organized   focused   positive   resilient
reliable   respectable   honest   confident   thoughtful   flexible
friendly   strong   creative   funny   attractive   loyal   hardworking
intelligent   kind   smart

Self-Care Scrabble Answer Key

1. IARALOTEXN _____ relaxation

2. BATEHRNIG ESSCEEXRI _____ breathing exercises

3. ITMEETDA _____ meditate

4. DEAR _____ read

5. WKAL _____ walk

6. SPLEE _____ sleep

7. GAYO _____ yoga

8. REECEXIS _____ exercise

9. CIAZLSIEO _____ socialize

10. ATBHE _____ bathe

11. CLORO _____ color

12. MFNRAIFTSAIO _____ affirmations

13. NETFEROICL _____ reflection

14. MCISU _____ music

15. UJRNLAO _____ journal

16. SUMNMAETE TITYVAIC _____ amusement activity

17. CKOO _____ cook

18. ASEMG _____ games

19. ELPUZZS _____ puzzles

20. GDENARGNI _____ gardening